Test Taking Techniques

Review and Resource Manual

by

Robin Donohoe Dennison, RN, MSN, CCRN, CCNS

&

Paulette D. Rollant, RN, MSN, PhD, CCRN

MAY 2002

Please direct your comments and/or queries to:
revmanuals@ana.org

The health care services delivery system is a volatile marketplace demanding superior knowledge, clinical skills, and competencies from all registered nurses. The *Test Taking Techniques Review and Resource Manual* was developed with the intent of helping nurses, whether still in school or preparing for licensure and certification exams, to master the skills required to take standardized tests.

The authors, editors, American Nurses Association (ANA), American Nurses Association's Publishing (ANP), American Nurses Credentialing Center (ANCC), and the Institute for Credentialing Innovation cannot accept responsibility for errors or omissions, or for any consequences or liability, injury, and/or damages to persons or property from application of the information in this manual and make no warranty, express or implied, with respect to the contents of the *Test Taking Techniques Review and Resource Manual.*

Published by:	Institute for Credentialing Innovation
The American Nurses Credentialing Center
8515 Georgia Ave., Suite 400
Silver Spring, MD 20910-3492
Phone: (301) 628-5000
www.nursecredentialing.org

ISBN-10: 1558101861
ISBN-13: 9781558101869

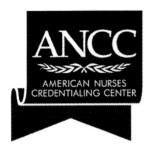

The mission of the American Nurses Credentialing Center is to promote excellence in nursing and health care globally through credentialing programs and related services.

To accomplish its mission, ANCC
- Certifies health care providers,
- Accredits educational providers, approvers, and programs,
- Recognizes excellence in nursing and health care services,
- Educates the public, and collaborates with organizations to advance the understanding of credentialing services, and
- Supports credentialing through research, education, and consultative services.

Taking a Certification Examination: Preparation and Performance

Robin Donohoe Dennison, RN, MSN, CCRN, CCNS
Paulette D. Rollant, RN, MSN, PhD, CCRN

I. **Why do you want to become certified?**
   A. #1 Reason: Self-satisfaction
      1. Validation of your knowledge of nursing within your chosen specialty
      2. This is the most commonly identified reason for taking this test
   B. Career mobility
      1. Certification through ANCC is a national credential; it is as prestigious in one state as another
   C. Promotion
      1. Certification is frequently a job requirement for advanced practice positions
      2. Certification is many times a critical requirement for promotion up a clinical career ladder
   D. Money
      1. Some hospitals offer a bonus for certification
      2. Some hospitals offer an hourly differential for certification
      3. Many hospitals reimburse the nurse for the expense of taking a certification examination if a passing score is attained

II. **Preparing for a certification examination**
   A. Be positive!
      1. "Since the mind is a specific biocomputer, it needs specific instructions and directions. The reason most people never reach their goals is that they don't define them, learn about them, or ever seriously consider them believable or achievable. Winners can tell you where they are going, what they plan to do along the way, and who will be sharing the adventure with them."
      Denis Waitley
      2. You've made it through nursing school and boards; this test is strictly for you!
         a. Write affirmations (positive statements)
         b. Record these on audiotape and play them over and over (to your brain)
         c. Examples of Affirmations

1) "I am an excellent test-taker."
2) "I am a knowledgeable specialist in ____ nursing."
3) "I will pass this test."
    3. Remember: "Decide what you want, decide what you are willing to exchange for it. Establish your priorities and go to work."
    H. L. Hunt
B. Prepare for the test
    1. Organize individual study or study groups
        a. Study groups may be particularly helpful for reviewing questions
        b. Choose study members wisely; do not choose members that are likely to not complete their assignment or consistently participate
    2. Review content areas
        a. Plan to review a system or content area per evening, day, or weekend, depending on how much time you have left before the examination
    3. Create memory joggers
        a. Memory jogger are frequently mnemonics such as "on old Olympus towering tops a Fin and German viewed some hops" for the names of the 12 cranial nerves
    4. Create recall associations
        a. Some of the best recall associations are actual patients that you made have had; for example, a patient with hypertriglyceridemia who developed pancreatitis, then developed acute respiratory distress syndrome (ARDS) as a complication, and, consistent with the high mortality of ARDS, the patient died
    5. Take a practice test at least 4 weeks before the examination; use this to identify weak areas for final study time
    6. Practice using your test-taking skills by doing lots of practice questions
        a. When checking your answer, always read the rationale
            1) The question on the exam may not be exactly like the practice question, but the concept may be tested
            2) Reading the rationale helps you learn the concept
        b. When checking your answer, ask yourself why you missed the question
            1) If you missed the question because you misread the question or one of the options, concentrate on slowing down and reading more thoughtfully

  2) If you missed the question because you lacked the necessary knowledge, identify the content as a weak area for more study

 C. Final preparations
  1. Don't cram the night before the exam
  2. Go to bed at a reasonable hour
  3. Avoid drugs or alcohol
  4. Choose to wear comfortable, layered clothes
  5. Eat a healthy but light meal before leaving to take the exam
   a. Avoid simple carbohydrates like a donut or Danish
   b. Choose to eat something with protein and fat to sustain you through the exam; examples include peanut butter on toast or an egg sandwich
  6. Don't forget your admission ticket and two forms of identification; at least one form of identification must have a photograph and signature
  7. Arrive at the site *at least* 15 minutes early
  8. Recite your affirmations on the trip to the examination site and maintain positive thoughts

III. Test-taking skills
 A. Mentally highlight key points as you read the question
  1. Age and gender of the patient
  2. Setting
   a. Acute care
   b. Primary care
   c. Home care
  3. Medical diagnosis and other coexisting diagnoses
  4. Timeframe in relation to admission, pain, trauma, surgery, etc.
   a. Immediately after
   b. Prior to
   c. Upon arrival
   d. During
   e. Initial day
   f. 3 days versus 7 days
 B. Look for key words like:
  1. Except, least or, never
  2. Indicated or contraindicated

3. Always
4. First or priority
5. Best

C. Read questions thoroughly
1. After you read the stem, answer the question without looking at the options
   a. You have probably been told, that if the answer that you come up with in your head after reading the question is among the four options, then it must be correct. PROBABLY but. . .
      1) Read ALL options as well as the stem
         a) There may be one better than your answer
         b) If you think option a is correct, jump down to option d and read the options in reverse
2. After reading the question
   a. Eliminate clearly wrong options to improve your odds for correct answer selection
   b. Eliminate similar options that say essentially the same thing
3. Identify if the question is asking about a global response or a specific item
   a. With some questions the more general or comprehensive option is a better answer than an option that is correct yet more specific or limited
   b. Choose the answer that matches the question in scope
      1) If it is a general question: give a general answer
      2) If it is a specific question: give a specific answer

D. Do not assume information that is not given
1. The only assumption is an ideal situation unless the question indicates otherwise
2. Remember
   a. All important information is included (if the patient is a diabetic, the question would indicate so)
   b. Included information is probably important (if the question indicates an amylase and lipase level, it is probably to rule in or out pancreatitis but it *may* be included as a distractor)

E. Answer easy questions first
1. Omit questions that you do not know the answer to but mark them to go back to if you have time.
   a. Before you run out of time, go back and fill in a choice
2. Don't leave any question blank

F. Answering priority questions

1. If I don't do this, my patient will die
    a. Always follow ABC: airway; breathing; circulation
2. If I don't do this, my patient will have serious complications or long-term sequelae
    a. Consider this as D: disability
3. If I don't do this, my patient will have pain or discomfort
    a. Consider acute pain as the #1 priority unless there is a life-threatening situation
    b. Choose narcotics for severe acute pain
4. ACTUAL problems always take precedence over *potential* problems
    a. If prioritizing between two potential problems, the priority is the one that is most life-threatening

G. Making decisions
1. If the question asks what to do next in a situation, use the nursing process to determine the next step
2. If the question asks what a patient needs, use Maslow's hierarchy of needs to determine the initial need
3. If the patient doesn't have an urgent physiologic need, focus on patient safety
4. Choose actions to check the patient first and equipment second
5. Look at the big picture and the organ systems involved; prioritize your assessment with the involved systems first
6. Pulmonary and cardiovascular systems are always the priority in any life-threatening situation
7. If all options are correct, prioritize by recalling well-known principles or theories or processes (e.g., Maslow's Hierarchy of Needs, Erikson's developmental tasks, Kubler-Ross' stages of death and dying, steps of the nursing process, principles of adult education)
8. Look for similar words used in the question and the options; if you find similar words, feelings, or behavior in the question and one of the options, it is probably the correct option

H. Guessing
1. Guessing should be used only when all else fails; you are not penalized for guessing
2. First eliminate any choices that you can; guess between two choices instead of four
3. Eliminate similar options since they could not both be correct

4. If you just have no idea, look for the different answer among the options
    a. Three antibiotics and an antifungal, choose the antifungal option
    b. Three beta-blockers and a calcium channel blocker, choose the calcium channel blocker option
    c. Three very specific and one very general option, choose the general or comprehensive option
    d. Etc.
I. Conserving mental energy
    1. The usual method of reading is to read the question in the order that it is written: case study, question, options
    2. What is frequently done though is to read the case study, question, reread case study, options
    3. Try this:
        a. Skip the case study
        b. Read the question
        c. Now read the case study
        d. Re-read the question
        e. Then read the options
        f. Though it is unlikely that you will run out of time taking the exam, you mental energy may be depleted
J. Maintaining concentration
    1. **C**hange your **P**rocess of **R**eading the case study, the question & the options
        a. Read the options in reverse order from option *d* to option *a*. Use this action especially when you suspect that option a or b is the correct option
        b. Make this change every 25 to 50 questions OR
            1) When you are physically tired, mentally anxious, or lose your concentration abilities
            2) When you come to the easier or the more difficult questions
    2. Rephrase the question rather than rereading the same question over and over
    3. Write down formulas, normal values, toxic levels, etc. on your scrape paper before you do the first question
    4. Use 3 S-L-O-W DEEP breaths to regroup and get re-focused at any time
    5. Take a mini-mental vacation after the harder questions
    6. Sign out and go to the restroom and splash water on your face if you are losing your ability to concentration

            a. Remember that the clock does not stop during this time so consider this if you are a slow test-taker
    K. Dealing with questions with multiple answers
        1. If the answer has more than one answer (such as x and y), both (or all) of the answers must be correct for the option to be correct
        2. These questions are usually written as a series of answers such option *a* is dog, cat, bird, option *b* is dog, cat, snake, option *c* is dog, bird, snake, and option *d* is cat, bird, snake; the correct option is the one that lists all three correct answers.
    L. Changing answers: know your pattern of errors
        1. If you tend to miss questions because you don't read them thoroughly and you realize that you misread this one question, then by all means change your answer
        2. If you tend to miss questions even though you read them thoroughly, don't change your initial answer
    M. Answering math questions
        1. Usually this is a drug calculation
            a. If this is a weak area for you, write down formulas on your scrap paper before you do question #1
            b. Recheck your math if you have time
            c. Calculators are not allowed
    N. Budgeting your time
        1. Time limit: 4 hours
            a. This is sufficient time to complete the test unless you are a very slow test taker
                1) Proceed quickly and carefully through the examination and do not spend an inordinate amount of time on individual questions

IV. More About the Test
    A. Consists of 175 items
        1. 150 graded items
        2. 25 test items; you will not know which ones are the test items
    B. Some tests are computerized and administered by Sylvian Prometric which can be scheduled when you want to take the exam and some tests are pencil and paper tests which are scheduled twice a year

V. Congratulations!
    A. For having the initiative to take this exam

B. Prepare, use your test-taking skills during the exam, and then sit back and wait for your passing score to arrive

VI. Selected References

A. Johnson S: *Taking the Anxiety Out of Taking Tests*, Oakland, CA, 1997, New Harbinger Publications, Inc.

B. Nugent P, Vitale B: *Test Success: Test-Taking Techniques for Beginning Nursing Students*, 2nd edition, Philadelphia, 1993, F. A. Davis Company.

C. Rollant P: *Soar to Success – Do Your Best on Nursing Tests!* St. Louis, 1999, Mosby.

D. Sides M, Korchek N: *Nurse's Guide to Successful Test-Taking*, Philadelphia, 1994, Lippincott.

VII. Practice Questions to Let You Practice These Test-Taking Skills!

1. One of the goals of a patient's care is that he remains free of infection. To evaluate if this goal has been met, the nurse would observe for:
   a. A change in the patient's complete blood counts.
   b. A normal body temperature.
   c. A change in the level of consciousness.
   d. A change in the patient's white blood cell count.

The answer is b.

Test-taking skill: The clue in options *a*, *c*, and *d* is the word 'change.' Note that the direction of the change is not stated. Thus, these options are not the best answer even though they sound good and are somewhat true statements. Also, if you had no idea of the answer, an approach you could have used is to cluster 3 similar options. This cluster would be options *a*, *c*, and *d* with the word 'change.' Then select the odd option out of the cluster, option *b*.

2. A nurse would expect a patient with pneumonia that has resolved to cough up sputum that is:
   a. Red or pink and frothy.
   b. Clear or white and thin.
   c. Brown or gray and smoky-smelling.
   d. Yellow or green and thick.

The answer is b.

Test-taking skill: If you selected option *d*, you have misread the question to ask about the findings of pneumonia. The question is asking about 'resolved pneumonia.' Thus, option *b* is the

correct answer. Option *a* has the clue 'frothy' which commonly indicates pulmonary edema. Option *c* reflects the results of an inhalation injury.

3. A patient is scheduled for a liver biopsy in two days. The pretest lab work has returned to the outpatient office. Which of these reports is a priority for the nurse to notify the physician about by the end of the day?
    a. Hemoglobin of 10.5 grams/dl
    b. Activated partial thromboplastin time of 45 second
    c. Elevated ALT and AST
    d. Elevated ammonia level

The answer is b.

Test-taking skill: If you are looking for an abnormal finding when you read the options, you discovered that all of the options are abnormal findings. You can anticipate that all of the options appear correct when the question has words like priority, initial, best, or first in it. So as you read the options think about significance. Then, refer to the clues in the stem. You know how vascular the liver is and that the major complication of 'liver biopsy' is bleeding. Therefore, the elevated aPTT is the priority.

4. Which roommate would you choose for a child with leukemia?
    a. A teenager with leukemia
    b. A child with suspected tuberculosis
    c. A toddler with intestinal inflammation
    d. A child with influenza

Test-taking skill: The initial decision to be made is: which is the priority? Is the age of the patient or the diagnosis more important in relation to the selection of a roommate? Many times the age is matched. However, the diagnosis of each patient is the priority in this question. The immunocompromise of the patient makes any other patient with infection or inflammation an unacceptable roommate.

5. A patient is admitted to an alcoholic treatment center. He reports drinking over a quart of liquor a day for 5 to 7 years. He has been drinking up until the time of admission. The orders include a regimen for a diet as tolerated, thiamine injection daily x 3, and a tranquilizer q 4 hours. Which of the following statement is correct?
    a. Delirium tremens will probably develop within the initial 24 hours of hospitalization.

b. Delirium tremens will probably develop between 48 and 72 hours of hospitalization.
   c. There is minimal risk of delirium tremens in this patient because he is receiving thiamine.
   d. This patient is unlikely to develop delirium tremors.

The answer is d.

Test-taking skill: If you selected option *c*, you have 2 problems. The first problem is misconception that thiamine prevents delirium tremens. The second problem is that you may have misread the second part of the option by thinking of another medication as you read the word, thiamine. Or you may have thought that the first part of this option was correct (and it is) and you then glossed over the second part of the option that is incorrect. This misreading 2 part options may be a chronic problem for you.

If you selected option *b*, the good news is that you have the knowledge that delirium tremens occur within 48 to 72 hours from the time of alcohol cessation. The bad news is that you omitted critical information in the stem that a tranquilizer was ordered for every 4 hours. This will minimize the risk of alcohol withdrawal. If you selected option *a*, you may have not focused on the clues in the stem including that the patient drank up until admission and that a tranquilizer was ordered.

Actions that will help you avoid the mistakes above are to change how you read the information, the question and the options. When there is a lot of information in the stem, read the question first. As you read this information, use your scrap paper to write a few notes as if you were taking a nursing report. Pay particular attention to the timeframes and types of medications. With 2 part options, once you have made your option selection, read the second part of the option first and the first part of the option last. Then you will catch any misreading of the given information.

6. The most important aspect to hand washing is which of these items?
   a. Soap
   b. Friction
   c. Paper towels
   d. Warm water

The answer is b.

Test-taking skill: In preparing for any test, be sure to review the basics. This is an easy question but it is a frequently missed question. Note that all of the options are correct and the question is

asking for the 'most important' aspect. These priority or "most important" questions are some of the most difficult ones on any test.

7. A mother has been caring for her infant with celiac disease. How can the nurse tell that the infant is being adequately nourished?
   a. By evaluating the infant's length and weight
   b. By evaluating the infant's score on the developmental chart
   c. By asking the mother what she thinks
   d. By having a 72 hour dietary recall completed by the mother

The answer is a.

Test-taking skill: The length of the infant is the same as the height in older children and adults. If you selected option *b*, your focus is too broad since the developmental chart includes height and weight and other developmental characteristics as motor, neurologic functioning, and thinking skills. Option *c* is subjective data, which is usually not the best answer in most situations unless it is combined with objective data. Most test-takers who select option *d* have really thought of a 24 hour recall as they read the option. As stated a 72-hour recall is subjective data with little credibility. Just think -- could you at this moment, write down what you have eaten in the last 3 days???

When assessment information is given in the options, label the data as subjective or objective. In this case, options *a* and *b* are objective data and options *c* and *d* are subjective data, which can usually be eliminated first. The second step is to compare the remaining options in light of their similarities and differences.

8. A patient is sent home on the medication Coumadin. The nurse is at highest risk for negligence in which of the following circumstances?
   a. The patient does not wear the medic alert band after discharge from the hospital.
   b. The nurse failed to document patient education regarding anticoagulant therapy.
   c. The patient did not show up for the second follow-up visit.
   d. The nurse did not call the physician's office the PT done the morning of the patient's discharge.

The answer is b.

Test-taking skill: If you selected options *a* or *c*, you have misread the question which focuses on the nurse. These options are focused on the patient. Option *d* sounds good but it does not state that the lab reports were abnormal. Therefore, it is not the best answer. If you selected option *b*, you are correct to recall that if it is not documented, it reflects that it was not done. Education is very important to safety for patients receiving anticoagulants.

9. A nurse would expect a patient with pneumonia to cough up sputum that is:
    a. Red or pink and frothy.
    b. Clear or white and thin.
    c. Brown or gray and smoky-smelling.
    d. Yellow or green and thick.

The answer is d.

Test-taking skill: Avoid thinking that the test has a repeat of the same question. The test may have similar questions such as this with a different question or time frame attached to it and with the options the same. The prior similar question was about resolved pneumonia. Other cautions – avoid reading into the information to think viral or bacterial pneumonia. This question is about findings of pneumonia in general.

10. A 21 year old patient with acute renal failure after hemorrhagic shock fails to respond to appropriate therapy to correct the renal failure. Urine output is 275 ml for 24 hours; creatinine is 7.2 mg/dl; and blood urea nitrogen is 90 mg/dl. Which of the following would the nurse expect to see as this patient progresses into a chronic renal failure?
    a. Anemia
    b. Hypokalemia
    c. Diaphoresis
    d. Hypotension

The answer is a.

Test-taking skill: It is helpful especially on questions with long stems to read the actual question first, then the case study, and finally all the options. In this case, you can make a selection without having to read the information in the stem. The question is 'which of the following is expected during progression into chronic renal failure?' The information in the stem is simply history of events leading up to the suspected chronic renal failure.

As you read the options, keep in mind the word 'chronic' as you focus on whether the option is a chronic or acute finding. Options c and d are more of an acute nature. Also, remember that patients with chronic renal failure tend to be hypertensive rather than hypotensive. So eliminate both of those options. To decide between the hypokalemia and anemia, think of what you know. In both acute and chronic renal failure, the most life-threatening electrolyte imbalance is hyperkalemia. Therefore, anemia is the correct answer.

If you answered option a, based on the information in the stem that the patient had hemorrhagic shock, you got the answer right for the wrong reason. The anemia of chronic renal failure is related to deficiency of erythropoietin, a hormone secreted by the kidney.

11. One of the goals of any patient's care is that he remain free of infection. Which of the following would indicate that this goal has not been met?
    a. An increase in urine output.
    b. No change in body temperature.
    c. A decrease in the level of consciousness.
    d. A increase in white blood cell count.

The answer is d.

Test-taking skill: Consider how specific each option is. The answer most specific to infection listed here is an increase in WBC. There is a change in level of consciousness with sepsis but not with infection. The body temperature would be expected to increase. No specific change in urine output would indicate infection.

12. What of the following is the best time for patients to take antacids?
    a. 30 minutes before meals
    b. 1 hour after meals
    c. On an empty stomach
    d. 2 hours after meals

The answer is b.

Test-taking skill: The action called 'clustering' or 'grouping' of 3 similar options will help you to select the correct answer. Options a, c and d are all the same instruction that is stated in a different way so the correct answer is option b. Taking antacids 1 hour after meals will be effective to reduce stomach acid for about 3 hours afterwards.

13. A middle aged Mexican-American patient refuses to eat the hospital prepared food and eats only flour tortillas, bean, and rice brought in by the family. Which of the following should the nurse be most concerned about?
    a. That the patient is consuming adequate nutrients and a balanced diet.
    b. That the patient is eating food provided by the dietary department.
    c. That the dietary department provide foods that the patient likes.
    d. That the patient is consuming adequate calories.

The answer is a.

Test-taking skill: Sometimes it is helpful to change your process for reading the options. Start at option *d* and read backwards to options *c*, then *b*, and then *a*. Try this technique when you are starting to find the process monotonous. With the use of this backward reading process, your mind will be more alert to compare the options as you read each. As you read each option, ask yourself if this is a true or false statement based on what the question asked. Option d is clearly wrong because he may eat plenty of calories with very little protein or vitamins. The focus should be on adequate nutrients and balance rather than just making sure that he eats (or the dietary department provides) the food. Option *a* is the most encompassing and correct of the options.

14. What of the following is the major problem that occurs with severe diarrhea?
    a. Fluid and electrolyte imbalance
    b. Spasmodic abdominal cramps
    c. Skin irritation of the anal region
    d. Disruption of lifestyle

The answer is a.

Test-taking skill: If you selected any option other than option *a*, you most likely misread the question. The clue is that the question asks for the 'major problem.' This should have signaled you to read the options with the intent to put them in order of priority. All of them are correct answers and you were to select the major problem.

If you read option *a*, selected it, and went on to the next question, you have a high risk of failing multiple choice tests. Questions with options that are all correct are commonly missed when all the options are not read. To prevent such an event from happening to you, do this. When you think that option *a* is correct, immediately jump to option *d* and read it. Then read options *c* then *b*. Reread option *a* and if you still think it is the best answer, select it.

15. In which of the following situations is a toddler at highest risk for lead poisoning?
    a. The toddler chews on the wood part of a #2 pencil.
    b. The family of the toddler lives next door to old apartments.
    c. The family of the toddler lives in an old house.
    d. The day care center where the toddler visits 3 times a week is located in a historic building.

The answer is c.

Test-taking skill: The clue in the question is 'at highest risk.' As you read the options you need to think in terms of frequency to the exposure. Option *c* reflects the more frequent exposure. If you selected option *a*, you misread the option. It states 'chews on the wood' rather the entire pencil and a #2 lead pencil does not contain lead. It contains graphite for the 'lead.' If you chose options *b* or *c* you focused on the words 'old' and 'historic' but did not consider the frequency of exposure.

16. 56-year-old woman is admitted with a diagnosis of bacterial pneumonia. Which of these findings would the nurse expect to see on the laboratory results?
    a. Elevated IgE levels
    b. Shift to the left in the WBC differential
    c. Hemoglobin of 10 gm/dl and HCT of 30%
    d. WBC count below 10,000 mm^3

The answer is b.

Test-taking skill: Since the diagnosis is an infection, one of the options related to WBC is most logical. Even if you don't know that a shift to the left indicates an increase in the number of bands seen in acute infection, you do know that a WBC below 10,000 is a normal value. Option *b* is the logical choice. Slow down, calm down, and be logical.

17. A patient has bacterial pneumonia as a result of *Staphylococcus aureus*. Which of these findings would you expect?
    a. Hyperresonance to percussion over the area
    b. Dullness to percussion over the area
    c. Resonance to percussion over the area
    d. Tympany to percussion over the area

The answer is b.

Test-taking skill: Pneumonia is not normal so eliminate option c which is a normal finding. Tympany and hyperresonance both indicate excessive air. Hyperresonance (option a) is noted over emphysematous lungs or pneumothorax and tympany (option d) is heard over the stomach and bowel. Consider that pneumonia is frequently referred to as consolidation and solid causes dullness to flatness on percussion. So choose option b.

18. The student nurse is assigned to a 42-year-old patient who has been admitted with the diagnosis of acute asthma attack. Which of these findings would the charge nurse want to review with the student as an expectation on this patient's laboratory results?
    a. An increased PaO_2
    b. A decreased hematocrit
    c. A decreased glucose level
    d. An increased eosinophil count

The answer is d.

Test-taking skill: If you selected option a, you have misread the question to be – what is the goal for the therapy? The question is -- what lab result is expected for a patient with acute asthma attack? It is frequently helpful to go through the options as true and false. Option a: false, the PaO_2 would go down not up. Option b: false, the hematocrit would be increased due to the significant dehydration caused by the tachypnea that occurs during acute asthma attack. Option c: false, the glucose may very well be increased related to sympathetic nervous system stimulation and stress response. Option d: true, since asthma is frequently triggered by allergic response and eosinophils are increased in allergic reactions.

19. Which of these antacids should be avoided with the diagnosis of hypertension?
    a. Tums
    b. Amphojel
    c. Maalox
    d. Rolaids

The answer is d.

Test-taking skill: Go with what you know. You know that patients with hypertension should avoid sodium. You know from TV commercials that Tums is high in calcium. Maalox is a magnesium antacid. Amphojel is an aluminum antacid. Rolaids is dihydroxyaluminum sodium carbonate and is high in sodium. It should be avoided for patients with hypertension.

20. Which of these is the most classic diagnostic finding with an acute episode of Ménière's disease?
   a. Severe prostrating vertigo with nausea and vomiting
   b. Feelings of fullness in the affected side of the head
   c. Unilateral recurrent tinnitus
   d. Intolerance to loud noises with hearing loss

The answer is a.

Test-taking skill: If you selected any option other than option *a*, you have missed the clues in the question of 'most classic diagnostic finding' and in the 'acute episode' situation. All of the other findings are found in the in Ménière's disease on an ongoing basis.

21. A postmenopausal patient talks with the nurse about vitamin B_{12} injections. Which of the following statements indicates a need for the nurse to clarify information?
   a. "The injections won't change the color of my stool."
   b. "I will need to come to the office for weekly injections."
   c. "I believe I will have more energy."
   d. "The substance from the stomach needed to absorb this vitamin from my food is no longer there."

The answer is b.

Test-taking skill: This is a negatively stated question. Rephrasing the question clarifies it. Which statement made by a patient would indicate misinformation about vitamin B_{12} injections. Option *b* is an incorrect statement since injections will need to be monthly not weekly.

22. A patient is prescribed lithium (Lithonate). Which of the following substances when taken in excess may cause problems with the serum lithium levels for the patient?
   a. Tums antacid
   b. Bananas
   c. Potato chips
   d. Chocolate chip cookies

The answer is c.

Test-taking skill: As you read the options, think about which electrolyte, mineral or other substance is the food item most closely associated with. Tums are high in calcium. Potato chips

are high in sodium. Bananas are high in potassium. Chocolate chip cookies are high in carbohydrates. Excess sodium may increase renal elimination of lithium and reduce lithium levels, so choose option c. The only serum drug levels typically tested on examinations are digoxin, lithium, aminophylline, and phenytoin.

23. The most important nurse responsibility to prevent complications during mannitol (Osmitrol) infusion is to:
    a. Position patients in a prone position with the use of a deep intramuscular technique.
    b. Include an in-line filter for the prevention of infusion of particulate matter.
    c. Monitor blood pressure every 15 minutes for one hour.
    d. Evaluate urine output for response to the mannitol.

The answer is b.

Test-taking skill: If you selected any other option than option b, you missed the clues in the question and the options. The clues in the stem are 'during …administration' and 'to prevent complications. The clue in option a is that IM injection is not an infusion. In option c and d to monitor and to evaluate are not actions for the prevention of complications. They are actions to detect complications or to evaluate effect. Option b is the only option that meets the criteria of the question and the given clues.

Restating the questions is frequently helpful. Perhaps something like this: "To prevent complications during IV mannitol, what is most important?"

24. A patient with heart failure is being monitored to evaluate the effectiveness of a dose of furosemide (Lasix). A change in which of the following parameters is most likely to be the earliest reflection that venous return to the heart is reduced?
    a. Central venous pressure
    b. Blood pressure
    c. SaO_2 by pulse oximetry
    d. Heart rate

The answer is a.

Test-taking skill: The question asks for the 'earliest' finding that the 'venous return' is different. Central venous pressure is a direct reflection of venous return to the heart. You would expect it to be decreased as a result of the diuresis caused by the furosemide. Heart rate and BP may reflect changes in venous return but indirectly and likely to be later findings. SaO_2 is a reflection of the

oxygen saturation of hemoglobin. As the degree of pulmonary edema is reduced, it would be expected to improve but it would be a late change.

25. A patient is diagnosed with schizophrenia. As his condition improves the nurse should:
   a. Offer a rigid schedule to provide him with structure.
   b. Offer two or three choices so as not to overwhelm him.
   c. Offer no choices because he is incapable of decision making.
   d. Offer him a range of choices so that he can select activities he is really interested in.

The answer is b.

Test-taking skill: Option *a* is the correct answer if the question asked about 'upon admission.' Option *d* is the correct answer if the question asked about 'upon or near the discharge date.' Option *d* introduces new information that the patient is incapable of decision making and is not the correct answer. The clue in the question is 'as his condition improves.' This makes the best answer to be option *b*.

The hidden time frames in questions may result in misreading the question and the options. Examples of hidden timeframes are words or phrases such as before, during, after, upon admission, as the condition improves, and upon or in readiness for discharge.

26. When a patient has auditory hallucinations, the nurse's best action is to tell the patient:
   a. that they don't exist.
   b. that he must prove the voices are real.
   c. to get involved in a unit-based activity.
   d. that the voices must be frightening.

The answer is d.

Test-taking skill: Option *d* is the correct action when a patient is psychotic or out of touch with reality as this patient is. It is appropriate to focus on their feelings rather than the actual hallucination. A psychotic patient should not be included in group activities such as option *c* suggests and they should not be challenged as in options *a* and *b*.

27. Which of the following is a side effect of the antipsychotic medication chlorpromazine HCl (Thorazine)?
   a. Nausea
   b. Drowsiness

c. Hypertension
   d. Frequent urination

The answer is b.

Test-taking skill: If you selected option *a*, you were thinking too general for the specific question about an antipsychotic medication. In general, nausea is a side effect of many drugs. The correct option is option *b*. Remember that with this drug classification the patient is advised to avoid alcohol ingestion which may increase the effects of the drowsiness.

If you selected option *c*, you may have misread this option to read "hypotension" instead of the word "hypertension" since you were thinking hypotension. Sometimes we see what we expect to see. Your thinking (hypotension) is correct. However, your reading of the actual word is incorrect. Is this a consistent problem for you? If you answered yes, then you need to stop and make extra effort on those hyper or hypo types of options.

If you selected option *d*, consider that there are very few drug classifications that result in frequent urination. They are the diuretics and the cholinergics.

28. The nurse would expect a patient with pulmonary edema to cough up sputum that is:
    a. Red or pink and frothy
    b. Clear or white and thin
    c. Brown or gray and sooty-smelling
    d. Yellow or green and thick

The answer is a.

Test-taking skill: If you selected any option other than option *a*, you have misread the question. You may have thought this was a repeat question since the options are exactly the same as a few questions given earlier. Beware of this type of situation and do not immediately answer the same option you did in the past. When you have these types of thoughts tell yourself to pay closer attention to what the question is about.

Another caution for those of you who knew the answer was option *a* and didn't read the other options. When you have the urge to make a choice and not read all of the options, do this. Jump down to the last option and read the options backwards from option *d* to *a*. This simple action will result in more focus with accurate decision-making skills.

29. A patient is to be discharged receiving scheduled doses of morphine sulfate by the intravenous route. The patient has been on this medication for 2 weeks while in the hospital. Which of these foods would be recommended to reduce the risk of a significant side effect of morphine?
   a. Rice cereal with whole milk
   b. Peanut butter sandwiches
   c. Bran cereal with 2% milk
   d. Cheese sandwiches

The answer is c.

Test-taking skill: The question requires 2 levels of thinking skills. First is to think that morphine is a narcotic analgesic with the side effect of constipation especially with long term use. The second level of thinking is to realize the question is asking what food aids in the prevention of constipation. Then you can use the cluster technique to group options a, b, and d into the group of food that have a tendency to cause constipation – whole milk, peanut butter and cheese.

The odd option out – 2% milk and bran is the correct answer. Keep in mind that bran is a bulk former and helps to prevent constipation when fluids and exercise requirements are met.

30. Which of the following foods would be discouraged or allowed only in limited amounts for a patient with renal failure?
   a. Apples
   b. Dried fruit
   c. Cranberries
   d. Apricots

The answer is d.

Test-taking skill: The major point here is renal failure. Now consider what is restricted. That would be fluids, potassium phosphorus, magnesium, and sodium. The potassium is the focus in this question in relation to the given food samples. Of the given foods, apricots have the highest potassium and need to be avoided. If you missed this question, it indicates that you need to review foods for high and low potassium content. This type of question may will be asked in a situation of renal failure and of the use of potassium losing diuretics.

31. Which of the following symptoms reported by a patient taking levothyroxine sodium (Synthroid) might indicate a subtherapeutic thyroid level?

a. chronic constipation
b. insomnia
c. palpitations
d. weight loss

The answer is a.

Test-taking skill: The correct option is option *a*. Persistent constipation would likely indicate that the medication is at a subtherapeutic level and would need to be increased. This may be a new type of question for you since the focus is on findings that indicate a need for more medication. Many questions ask for findings associated with overdosage or adverse effect.

Another important clue is the direction of change of the options. Constipation is a hypo effect while insomnia, palpitations, and weight loss could be indicative of hyperthyroidism rather than hypothyroidism.

Also, this is a multi-level thinking question. First you have to associate the medication with thyroid function. This is easy since the last part of Synthroid is like 'thyroid.' Then you have to think of the problems with too much or too little of the medication. Recall that thyroid hormones influence most of the body systems through the effect on metabolism.

32. Which of the following aspects of aging increases the risk of injury that needs to be reinforced to the ancillary staff?
    a. Decreased lung compliance
    b. Decrease visual acuity and altered proprioception
    c. Decreased peristalsis
    d. Decreased cardiac contractility

The answer is b.

Test-taking skill: All answers are correct if the question is just about the physical effects of aging. However, injury is most likely to occur with physical movement so choose the option associated with locomotion.

33. Which lunch menu would be most helpful for your postoperative patient for wound healing?
    a. A one egg Spanish omelet
    b. A baked potato with sour cream
    c. Lemon chicken and brown rice

    d. Tomato stuffed with cottage cheese

The answer is c.

Test-taking skill: First think about the most important nutritional considerations for wound healing. That would be protein, vitamin C, zinc. Option c has protein in the chicken and the rice and vitamin C. Options a and d have protein and vitamin C (tomato) but c has more protein. Option b is the lowest in protein and vitamin C.

34. If you saw a nurse colleague perform all of these actions, which one would require that report the action to the charge nurse?
    a. Auscultate lung sounds using the bell of the stethoscope
    b. Give atropine for sinus tachycardia
    c. Give an IM injection with a one inch 25 gauge needle
    d. Withdraw Humulin-N insulin after shaking the bottle

The answer is b.

Test-taking skill: You should have expected that all actions are inappropriate but your task is to put them in priority from the greatest to the least harmful. The best approach is to ask yourself: "which of these actions would likely have the most harmful outcome?" Option b is the correct answer since atropine will increase the heart rate and the patient is already in sinus tachycardia. Atropine is given for sinus bradycardia, sinus arrest, or AV block. If you selected options a or d, note that both are not correct technique but are unlikely to harm the patient.

If you selected option c, you are on the right track to think that the medication might not go through the needle or the patient may be obese and the medication will not go into the muscle. However, look back to the options. None of that information is included. Thus, if you thought that and chose option c, you have read into the option.

35. Which of these patients is it most appropriate for the charge nurse to assign to the patient care assistant?
    a. A patient who needs a dressing change
    b. A patient who has returned from an X-ray procedure
    c. A patient with a two hour turning schedule
    d. A patient to be discharged that day

The answer is c.

Test-taking skill: If you narrowed the options to *b* and *c*, you have identified that options *a* and *d* require a higher level of skill from a licensed staff member. To decide between options *b* and *c* ask the question: "Which patient would be the more stable?" Option *c* is the correct answer. The patient in option *b* has more potential to be unstable since the type of X-ray procedure is not given.

36. A patient with severe COPD needs to have a liver biopsy. How would you position the patient for the procedure?
    a. A right side lying position with the knees straight
    b. A left side lying position with the knees slightly bent
    c. A dorsal recumbent with the right arm behind the head and a low fowler's bed position
    d. A dorsal recumbent with the right arm behind the head and a very low fowler's bed position

The answer is c.

Test-taking skill: The two major clues are the timeframe 'for the procedure' and the preexisting problem (COPD). If you selected option *b*, it indicates that you need to review different procedures and the required positions. If you selected option *a*, perhaps you were thinking of a post liver biopsy position.

If you narrowed it down to options *c* and *d* you are on the right track. If you selected the correct answer, option *c*, you noted that the patient had a 'severe' lung problem. Thus, the higher position would be preferred. If you instead chose option *d*, you may have missed the clue in the stem identifying the severe COPD.

37. If planning care for a patient with acute asthma, the nurse should consider that patients diagnosed with asthma:
    a. should minimize fluid intake.
    b. have asthma attacks brought on by anxiety.
    c. may have difficulty coughing up sputum.
    d. will improve quickly with hospitalization.

The answer is c.

Test-taking skill: If you selected option *a*, you may have misread the option to read 'maximize' fluid intake since that is an appropriate action for persons with asthma. Patients with asthma have greater insensible loss of fluid by the respiratory tract because of tachypnea. Avoid absolute

options such as option *b*. Option *b* reads as if all asthma attacks are brought on by anxiety, which is a false statement.

Option *c* is the correct answer and is applicable to any patient with asthma. The dehydration that occurs causes thick, sticky mucus. Option *d* is a false statement. If you chose this option your thought is too narrow of a focus. Also, this is another example of an absolute statement where the intent is that 'all' patients with asthma improve quickly. This is a false statement.

38. In helping a mother set goals for her baby's care, the nurse should plan to emphasize the need for the mother to:
    a. learn about proper baby care.
    b. plan time to budget the finances.
    c. find a place to live.
    d. identify community resources.

The answer is a.

Test-taking skill: The immediate priority is to care how to care for the baby. The other issues are important but the baby's care is the focus.

39. In planning care for a 6 year old, the nurse should consider his development to recognize that:
    a. the child needs to be like his peers.
    b. separation anxiety is at its peak.
    c. a need for increased privacy exists.
    d. the fear about his body changing is greater than his fear of being apart from his parents.

The answer is c.

Test-taking skill: With the selection of option *a* or *d*, you may have been thinking of teenagers. For option *b*, a common error is to read this as "the preschool or school age child will have separation anxiety". That is correct thinking. However, the option states that separation anxiety is at its *peak*. Thus, this option is incorrect. Peak separation anxiety occurs in the toddler years. School age children like to have their physical privacy as compared to the preschooler or toddler so *c* is the correct option.

40. When is involutional depression most common?
    a. in women before age 45

b. in men age 50 to 60
c. in persons with a poor adjustment to middle age
d. following the endocrine changes of menopause

The answer is c.

Test-taking skill: Knowledge of involutional depression is not needed to answer this question correctly. First note that the question is a general question. Thus, the best option will be one of a general focus.

As you read the options, note that options *a*, *b*, and *d* are specific to men or women. These can be clustered under the umbrella of specific groups. Option *c* is the odd option since it is more general of a focus for persons. Thus, make an educated guess to select option *c*.

41. One hour after receiving a pain medication, a patient was still complaining of severe leg pain. The pain medication cannot be given again for another two hours. There is no change in the physical appearance of the leg, pulses are palpable, and the leg is warm. Which of the following is the most appropriate action by the nurse to help the patient deal with the pain?
    a. offer a magazine to read or turn on the relaxation channel on the TV
    b. close the door and guide the client in slow, rhythmic breathing techniques
    c. turn the lights down low, give the patient a back rub, and close the door
    d. call the physician to increase the dosage of the PRN medication

The answer is d.

Test-taking skill: If you chose option *a*, *b*, or *c*, you have missed the clue in the stem of 'severe' pain an hour after the pain medication was given. The actions in these three options are appropriate for mild or moderate pain. Severe pain usually requires higher doses of medication or a change of the type of medication.

42. Which is the most comprehensive definition for the nursing process?
    a. it is a nursing approach to medical diagnoses
    b. it is the method by which conceptual frameworks for nursing are put into practice
    c. it is a problem solving method which includes five steps of assessing, diagnosing, planning, intervening, and evaluating
    d. assessment is the first step in the nursing process

The answer is c.

Test-taking skill: The only option that is clearly wrong is option *a*. While options *b* and *d* are all correct, option *c* is the most comprehensive.

43. A nurse is caring for a patient with a colostomy. Which statement made by the patient indicates no need for additional teaching regarding when the pouch needs emptied?
    a. "I'll empty it prior to meals"
    b. "I'll empty it whenever it has feces or flatus in it"
    c. "I'll empty it daily at the same time"
    d. "I'll empty it whenever it is one third to one half full"

The answer is d.

Test-taking skill: If you chose options *a*, *b*, or *c*, you missed the clue that they are absolute statements. With the use of common sense, you would realize that the actions in these options would be impractical to implement consistently. Thus, only option left is option *d*, which is correct.

44. Which patient is at most risk for bladder cancer?
    a. a man who smoked for many years
    b. a man who is 50 years old
    c. a woman with endometriosis
    d. a woman who has bleached her hair blonde

The answer is a.

Test-taking skill: The clue in the stem is "at most risk." Of the given options, the person who has the greatest cancer risk is the smoker. Statistics suggest that if a person has one risk or has cancer, it puts them at a higher risk for other types of cancer.

If you selected option *b*, you chose an option that is too narrow with only age being the consideration. Endometriosis, the growth of endometrial tissue outside the uterus, has the problem of infertility rather than cancerous growths so eliminate option *c*. If you chose option *d* because of the colored hair, part of your thinking is correct. The dye has to be from the indigo plant – aniline dyes for dying the hair black is considered to be a risk for cancer of the bladder.

45. A woman in active labor is on the way to the hospital. What should the nurse do first once the patient is placed in the bed?
    a. check the vital signs

    b. get a urine sample
    c. check the cervix
    d. evaluate the intensity of contractions

The answer is c.

Test-taking skill: If you selected options *a* or *b*, you have missed the point that the woman is in active labor. Though all of the actions are appropriate, checking the cervix is most important.

With the selection of option *d*, you have misread the option to read to time the 'frequency' rather then 'intensity' of the contractions. This is an indication that you need to screen your thinking versus what is actually on the page. If you made this error here, you probably have a tendency to do this frequently on tests especially with content that you are familiar with from your clinical experience. Many times the easier questions are missed simply from misreading the options. You may have a tendency to see what you expect instead of what is actually there.

46. Which of these patients in the emergency department should the nurse check first?
    a. A patient in the manic state
    b. An elderly man with suspected organic brain syndrome
    c. A toddler with a black eye
    d. A teenager with singed facial hair

The answer is d.

Test-taking skill: If you selected options *a*, *b*, or *c*, you missed the association of singed facial hair with the exposure to heat or fire with the risk of smoke inhalation injury to the respiratory tract. The clue is that the question asked for a priority. Think airway.

47. A multipara woman arrives at the clinic with generalized complaints. Which action should the nurse do first?
    a. take the vital signs
    b. get a urine sample
    c. obtain the antepartal history
    d. check the cervix

The answer is a.

Test-taking skill: This question is a chance for you to read the question and to fight question hangover from a recent prior question. The correct answer is to take the vital signs. If you chose options *b*, *c*, or *d* you have read into the situation that the woman was pregnant.

Or you may have been thinking of the prior question in which the woman was in labor and the options were similar. Based on the given information, the woman is a multipara with generalized complaints. The measurement of vital signs is the first action to take.

48. Which of the following would be the priority for a patient with multiple trauma?
    a. open the airway
    b. set the fractured femur
    c. apply pressure to scalp laceration
    d. stabilize the cervical spine

The answer is a.

Test-taking skill: In any life-threatening situation, always follow A (airway), B (breathing), C (circulation), and D (disability). Opening the airway if the #1 priority (A), pressure on the scalp laceration (C) would be next, then stabilizing the cervical spine (D) would be next. Setting the fractured femur is the lowest priority.

49. Your patient is dying of cancer with metastasis to the brain. He has asked you not to allow his sister to visit. Today he is unconscious. His sister calls the unit crying and requests that she be allowed to visit. What is the most appropriate response?
    a. Gently explain that it was the patient's wish for her not to visit.
    b. Tell her that she will have to have the physician's permission to visit.
    c. Let her visit for a few minutes.
    d. Let her sit at the bedside for as long as she needs.

The answer is a.

Test-taking skill: The patient's needs and desires should always be honored if they are known even when he is incapacitated. You may also notice that options *b*, *c*, and *d* all may allow the sister to visit. Choose the one that is different, option *a*.

50. While bathing a 42 year old man admitted with an acute MI, he tells you that he is HIV-positive. Which of the following is the most appropriate action?
    a. Ask him how he contracted the virus

b. Flag his name outside his room and his chart with an HIV+ sticker
c. Tell his wife
d. Discuss prevention of transmission of the virus

The answer is d.

Test-taking skill: Obviously you need to respect his privacy so eliminate options *b* and *c*. Discussing methods of prevention of transmission of the virus (option *d*) is appropriate. Asking him how he contracted the virus (option *a*) is inappropriate.

Test-taking skill: When you think a question is difficult, regroup and refocus your thinking to look if you are adding information in your mind. Close your eyes. Take a deep breath. Then open your eyes to reread the question with a fresh mind. Then, read the options in reverse order from your original read. All the while, continue to identify clues in the question or the options. The result will be an identification of where you read into the question or the options. You will select the best answer based on the given information and not what you think was given.

American Nurses Association of Nursing Continuing Education Reviewers

Madeline K. Kiger, MS, RN, CS, PNP
Burleson, TX

Carolyn Blyth, MSN, RN
Picayune, MS

Michael Suraci
Annandale, VA

LuJaunna Walker, MSN, RN, CS
Fort Washington, MD

The Test Taking Techniques Review and Resource Manual is designed to meet the following objectives:

1. Identify key test taking strategies.
2. Formulate study plan based on your study needs.
3. Utilize the principles and rationale for effecting test taking.

For further information about ANCC's continuing education and review courses, please visit www.nursecredentialing.org.